HOW BLOOD WORKS

All You Need To Know About Blood Type and Health

Dr. Joseph U. Charlse

Table of Contents

CHAPTER I

Preface

About 2 billion humans globally are anemic, and nearly as many suffer from iron deficiency without anemia. Many don't even know they have it, simply feeling worn-out, torpid, and "foggy-headed." Sound familiar? Over six hundred million greater be afflicted by acute or from time to time unrecognized continual blood loss from causes which include heavy menstrual bleeding, obstetric hemorrhage, gastrointestinal bleeding, surgical procedure, and trauma. Anemia, iron deficiency, and bleeding are signs of "blood failure" and have primary bad fitness results. Blood Works, with contributions from forty eight leading international medical experts, is a ought to have book for all who need to appearance after their blood fitness.

Your blood is the essential fluid that continues you alive. Yet, whilst many of us recognize our ldl cholesterol stage and blood pressure, few people are aware about our blood be counted. What we don't recognize can affect our regular excellent of lifestyles and positioned us at hazard if we have bleeding, an injury, or require hospitalization.

Blood, and the vessels that comprise it, make up the biggest organ machine in the body. Its stability and fitness have to be maintained. For many years, the remedy of first inn for anemia and blood loss has been blood transfusion, which is largely a "liquid organ" transplant from some other character. In heart failure or kidney failure, organ transplantation is not first-line remedy. In blood failure, blood "transplantation" need to now not be the primary thing we reach for. Since the Nineteen Nineties, medical research has proven that the common use of blood transfusion isn't always the only remedy in many medical situations. It has been recognized as one of the maximum overused remedies in present day medicine, costing billions of greenbacks, while causing adjustments inside the recipient's immune gadget which could boom the hazard of headaches and death. In October 2021, the World Health Organization called for the pressing global implementation of Patient Blood Management (PBM), declaring "our personal blood remains the great issue to have in our veins."

CHAPTER II

Discussion on Blood

Blood is a combination of plasma, platelets, and red and white blood cells that circulate through the body. It elements essential materials, along with sugars, oxygen, and hormones, to cells and organs, and removes waste from cells.

Hematologists work to pick out and prevent blood and bone marrow sicknesses. They also study and treat the immune machine, blood clotting, and blood vessels.

Health situations that affect the blood can be existence threatening, but effective remedy is often available. In America, blood sicknesses accounted for 10,066Trusted Source deaths in 2008, commonly distinctive forms of anemia.

The Primary Additives Of Blood Are:

- Plasma

- Red blood cells

- White blood cells

- Platelets

Plasma

Plasma debts for around 55% of blood fluid in people. Plasma is 92% water, and the contents of the final 8% encompass:

- Glucose

- Hormones

- Proteins

- Mineral salts

- Fats

- Vitamins

The last 45% of blood specifically consists of red and white blood cells and platelets. Each of those has a critical role to play in preserving the blood functioning successfully.

Find out what plasma donation includes.

Red Blood Cells, Or Erythrocytes

Red blood cells have a slightly indented, flattened disk form. They delivery oxygen to and from the lungs. Hemoglobin is a protein that consists of iron and consists of oxygen to its destination. The existence span of a red blood cell is 4 months, and the body replaces them regularly. The human body produces around 2 million blood cells every 2d.

The predicted variety of red blood cells in a single drop (microliter) of blood is four.5–6.2 million in men and four.0–5.2 million in women.

White Blood Cells, Or Leukocytes

White blood cells make up much less than 1% of blood content material, forming important defenses against sickness and infection. The range of white blood cells in a microliter of blood normally stages from 3,700–10,500. Higher or lower ranges of white blood cells can suggest disease.

Platelets, Or Thrombocytes

Platelets interact with clotting proteins to save you or stop bleeding. There ought to be between 150,000 and 400,000 platelets in step with microliter of blood.

Bone marrow produces purple blood cells, white blood cells, and platelets, and from there they input the bloodstream. Plasma is normally water this is absorbed from ingested food and fluid by using the intestines. The coronary heart pumps them across the body as blood by using way of the blood vessels.

Functions

Blood has diverse features that are valuable to survival. They consist of:

- supplying oxygen to cells and tissues

- providing vital nutrients to cells, inclusive of amino acids, fatty acids, and glucose

- casting off waste substances, such as carbon dioxide, urea, and lactic acid

- Defensive the body from illnesses, infections, and overseas our bodies through the action of white blood cells

- regulating body temperature

The platelets in blood permit the clotting, or coagulation, of blood. When bleeding takes place, the platelets organization collectively to create a clot. The clot forms a scab, which stops the bleeding and allows defend the wound from infection.

CHAPTER III

How Antigens Determine Your Blood Type

No count number your kind, all blood incorporates the equal basic building blocks. Blood consists of red blood cells that transport oxygen, white blood cells that combat infections, and platelets that resource in clotting whilst you're injured. Plasma, a fluid that includes proteins and salts, incorporates all blood cells through your veins.

Your antigen make-up is the key component in determining your blood kind. Antigens reside at the surface of your pink blood cells, in which they serve as integrated safety gadgets on your blood deliver. These substances are designed to become aware of foreign cells and trigger immune responses that produce antibodies within the plasma to assault ability invaders.

The presence or absence of antigens on your red blood cells and corresponding antibodies for your plasma defines your ABO blood organization. This blood grouping device has four kinds:

- Group A: This blood group has A antigens and B antibodies.

- Group B: This blood group has B antigens and A antibodies.

- Group AB: This blood organization has A and B antigens and no antibodies.

- Group O: This organization doesn't have either A or B antigens, however it has each A and B antibodies.

This blood institution device can also appear honest, but it's still pretty new. In reality, Austrian doctor Karl Landsteiner found the life of antibodies and antigens in blood just over a century ago, in

1901. His work later caused the creation of blood groups, earned him a Nobel Prize in 1930, and contributed to great advances in medication.

The Rhesus System and Your Blood Type

A decade after receiving his Nobel Prize, Landsteiner and colleague A.S. Weiner located a secondary protein that still has a chief impact on blood kind. Their paintings with rhesus monkeys caused the introduction of the Rhesus device, which highlights the presence or absence of the Rh thing.

If your red blood cells have this protein, your plasma certainly includes Rh antigens. That way you're considered superb, or Rh+. If you don't have this protein, your blood is taken into consideration Rh-, or terrible.

Standard blood typing combines the ABO device with the Rhesus system to create an extra complete photograph of your blood profile. That means you can have certainly one of 8 blood types:

•	Type A+: Contains A and Rh antigens in addition to B antibodies.

- Type A-: Contains A antigens as well as B antibodies.

- Type B+: Contains B and Rh antigens as well as A antibodies.

- Type B-: Contains B antigens in addition to A antibodies.

- Type AB+: Contains A, B, and Rh antigens but no antibodies.

- Type AB-: Contains A and B antigens.

- Type O+: Contains Rh antigens in addition to A and B antibodies.

- Type O-: Contains no antigens however has A and B antibodies.

Although maximum humans have one of the 8 common blood types, a few humans don't match neatly into this fashionable machine. Over six hundred other antigens can are living on red blood cells, main to endless uncommon blood sorts. Since blood kind is hereditary, rare blood sorts generally exist in ethnic businesses.

CHAPTER IV

Why Blood Typing Is Important

Each blood kind includes a sensitive balance of antigens and antibodies, and no longer all blood sorts are well suited with each other. Since antibodies are designed to fight corresponding antigens, a transfusion that mixes incompatible blood sorts could purpose the antibodies in a single to assault the antigens in some other. These antibody attacks can result in agglutination, or the advent of clumps of purple blood cells. Agglutination can create clogs, stop circulate, and may purpose purple blood cells to cut up and leak, which triggers toxic reactions.

Since blending incompatible kinds may be dangerous or even deadly, know-how your blood kind is vital, especially in case you're donating blood or receiving a transfusion from a donor. After all, a few blood sorts can't pair thoroughly with others, while others are compatible with several other types. The 8 general blood corporations can pair as follows:

•	Type A+: Can donate blood to types A+ and AB+. Can acquire blood donations from types A+, A-, O+, and O-.

•	Type A-: Can donate blood to sorts A+, A-, AB+, and AB-. Can acquire blood donations from kinds A- and O-.

•	Type B+: Can donate blood to sorts B+ and AB+. Can receive blood donations from sorts B+, B-, O+, and O-.

•	Type B-: Can donate blood to types B+, B-, AB+, and AB-. Can obtain blood donations from kinds B- and O-.

- Type AB+: Can donate blood to kind AB+. Can get hold of blood donations from all 8 types.

- Type AB-: Can donate blood to sorts AB+ and AB-. Can acquire blood donations from sorts AB-, A-, B-, and O-.

- Type O+: Can donate blood to types O+, A+, B+, and AB+. Can receive blood donations from sorts O+ and O-.

- Type O-: Can donate blood to all eight types. Can acquire blood donations most effective from kind O-.

Overall, sorts O+ and A+ are with the aid of some distance the most commonplace blood types inside the United States, performing in 37 and 36 percentage of the populace, respectively. Almost 9% of Americans have both kind B+ or O- blood, while 6% have kind A-, and three% have type AB+ blood. Types B- and AB- are the least commonplace inside the U.S., performing in 2% and much less than 1% of the population, respectively.

What Your Blood Type May Tell You

While blood typing is crucial before a transfusion or a donation, expertise your blood kind also can screen plenty extra approximately you. Knowing your blood kind assist you to learn about your history and genetic make-up as well as your danger elements for developing severe fitness problems within the future.

Since every blood kind appears in various frequencies throughout the globe, expertise your blood kind should help you pinpoint your ancestors. For instance, blood kind Rh+ could be very not unusual throughout the globe. It tends to seem maximum often in Asia and Australia, however Western Europeans and those with Basque history have a number of the very best frequencies of blood type Rh-.

In addition, blood kind A appears often in all populations, however it's most foremost in North America and Europe. Blood type O is also not unusual round the sector, but it seems most often in Central and South America. In contrast, blood type B is notably uncommon out of doors of Central Asia, Northern India, and Russia.

In many instances, your blood type also can shed light on sicknesses to which you may be greater prone, as well as fitness conditions to which your body can be more resistant. After all, kind A is the oldest of the ABO blood businesses, whilst sorts O and B appeared a great deal later. Like most genetic mutations, blood types O and B gave bearers choose blessings, consisting of resistance to positive diseases.

While few studies have established clean links among blood kind and danger element for illnesses, several reports have suggested connections between the two. For instance, humans with blood kind AB have a tendency to have higher ranges of a protein that encourages blood clotting and can result in strokes. Along the identical strains, studies have proven that people with kind A and type B blood have a greater chance of developing type 2 diabetes.

In assessment, people with blood type O tend to have a extra resistance to many serious diseases. Several research have demonstrated that those with blood type O have a natural safety towards one of the most harmful types of malaria, while tests have additionally shown that people with blood type O actually have a considerably decreased danger of developing stomach most cancers. Studies have also shown that people with blood kind O have the lowest chance of developing cardiovascular ailment, suggesting that they will have obviously low degrees of inflammation and low-density lipoprotein (LDL) cholesterol.

CHAPTER V

What Influences Your Blood Type

Blood kind is a hereditary trait, as dad and mom' blood types decide their youngsters'. While children's blood types aren't always a precise match for one of their parents, knowledge parents' blood kinds can assist slim down the ability sorts that youngsters should have.

A single gene determines ABO blood kind, and 3 variations of the gene exist: A, B, and O. Both A and B versions of the blood kind gene are dominant, and the O version is recessive. Children inherit one model of the gene from every parent, ensuing in six potential combinations of genes that location them in considered one of 4 ABO businesses.

For instance, a baby who inherits an A model of the gene from one parent and a B version from the opposite could have blood type AB. Inheriting an A model and an O model of the gene will result in blood kind A, while inheriting two

O versions of the gene will bring about blood type O.

A separate gene determines whether kids have the Rh aspect. Since Rh element is either tremendous or poor, simplest two variations of this gene exist. In this case, the fantastic model is dominant, and the bad model is recessive. That way inheriting a wonderful version and a bad model of the gene will result in blood kind Rh+, while inheriting two terrible variations will result in blood type Rh-.

Although growing a hereditary chart can help in assessing

potential blood kind alternatives for contemporary and future generations, this approach isn't clinical. Only a reliable test can confirm your blood type.

How Blood Typing Is Done

To discover your blood kind, you'll need to provide a blood sample. To start the system, a clinician will sanitize your skin, make sure that your veins are seen, and then use a needle to draw a blood pattern. The clinician will then region gauze over the puncture region and proceed with checking out.

To complete the blood kind check, the clinician will divide your pattern into separate vials. The clinician will then blend your pattern with a solution that carries A and B antibodies. If your blood cells react by way of forming clumps, then your blood carries at the least one of the antigens. Next, the clinician will mix your plasma with either type A or kind B blood to decide whether your blood has A, B, or both antibodies. Finally, the clinician will use a comparable process of mixing your blood cells and plasma with Rh+ blood to decide your Rh aspect.

After this take a look at, you'll realize each your Rh factor and your ABO blood group, revealing your blood kind. Since most blood kind tests take mere minutes and the dangers are minimal, blood typing is a easy and cheaper process that may be notably informative.

Blood Type and Donation Needs

From sickle mobile patients who need recurring blood transfusions in the course of their lives and most cancers sufferers who require blood at some stage in a chain of chemotherapy remedies to sufferers of automobile injuries who need huge amounts of blood urgently, a person in the U.S. Desires a blood donation each seconds.

Although almost seven million U.S. Residents donate blood each yr., much less than 10% of humans eligible to donate achieve this. Since pink blood cells expire within six weeks of donation and platelets expire in just 5 days, blood donations are in consistent call for throughout the kingdom.

While red blood cells are in finest demand, many patients want plasma and platelets, too. Since blood kind O is well matched with the widest style of blood types, it has a tendency to be maximum regularly requested. Although nearly half of Americans have type O blood, kind O- is one of the least common amongst U.S. Citizens.

That manner this noticeably compatible blood kind has a tendency to be in quick deliver. Fortunately, giving blood is highly simple for eligible donors who can supply complete blood each eight weeks. Because a single donation can save up to three lives, giving blood can have a widespread impact, irrespective of what your blood type.

Whether you want to put together for a capacity clinical emergency, understand how your blood type should affect future children, determine your danger stage for sure diseases, or analyze more about hereditary elements, your blood kind has the solutions.

Blood Type and Organ Donation

If you want a new organ or you want to donate an organ, blood type trying out can assist assess your eligibility? The kidney donation process starts with blood typing, which determines the types of recipients who're well suited with you. Donors and recipients commonly in shape as follows:

Type A: Donors are compatible with kind A and AB recipients.

Type B: Donors are compatible with type B and AB recipients.

Type AB: Donors are well suited with kind AB recipients.

Type O: Donors are well suited with all recipients.

Next, each the donor and the recipient go through tissue typing, which compares 12 antigens to determine how compatible the tissue sorts are. While identical twins, siblings, parents, and kids have the fine probabilities of matching, even entire strangers may have few or maybe o mismatches.

Both patients also undergo a 2d tissue type check that assessments for antibodies that can attack the tissue. Since antibody ranges can trade over the years, maximum transplant recipients entire common tests for months after surgery.

In maximum instances, close household and exact blood type suits are perfect and increase the possibilities of fulfillment from an organ donation. However, antibody remedies may additionally allow recipients to obtain organs from donors without compatible blood kinds, in the long run increasing the range of donors available to a recipient in want of a transplant.

Knowing Your Blood Type

Many human beings recognize that knowing your blood type is critical inside the occasion you need a blood transfusion. But it could also be critical in different health scenarios.

CHAPTER VI

Disorders

Disorders and diseases of the blood can impair the numerous features that blood plays.

Some common blood disorders are:

• Anemia: This takes place while low pink blood mobile or hemoglobin levelsTrusted Source suggest the cells do now not transport oxygen efficiently, main to fatigue, faded skin, and other signs and symptoms.

- Blood clotting: Clotting facilitates wounds and accidents heal, however blood clots that form interior a blood vessel can create a blockage, which can be existence threatening. If clots become dislodged and circulate thru the coronary heart to the lungs, a pulmonary embolism can shape.

- **Blood Cancers:** Cancers which include leukemia, myeloma, and lymphoma occur whilst blood cells start to divide uncontrollably without demise off on the cease of their life cycle.

- **Hemophilia:** If someone has low tiers of clotting elements inside the blood, they are able to bruise or bleedTrusted Source very without problems. They might also bleed for too long after a minor harm or surgical treatment, or at some stage in menstruation. It impacts around 18,000 in the U.S.

- **Sickle Cellular Disease:** An inherited trait reasons purple blood cells to tackle a crescent shape. It affects over 100,000Trusted Source people in the U.S., commonly Black Americans. It can critically impact how blood capabilities and may be life threatening.

- **Thalassemia:** This is likewise a type of inherited anemia in which the body produces an uncommon shape of hemoglobin. It affected round 1,000Trusted Source humans in the U.S. In 2008 and is most commonplace in humans from across the Mediterranean and elements of Asia.

If signs recommend a person might also have a blood ailment, they need to seek scientific recommendation. A physician may refer them to a specialist in blood problems, referred to as a hematologist.

Blood is critical for maintaining the health and lifestyles of the human frame. It has many functions, which includes handing over vitamins and oxygen. The 4 primary components of blood are purple blood cells, white blood cells, plasma, and platelets.

Problems that get up because of infection or blood loss may be lifestyles threatening, but powerful remedy is to be had for lots blood-associated issues.

CHAPTER VII

What Happens to Donated Blood?

Step One: The Donation Process

The donor completes the registration procedure.

The donor gives a medical history and undergoes a mini bodily examination.

Blood is donated. The Red Cross collects numerous check tubes and one pint of blood from the donor.

Identical barcoded labels are positioned at the donor's file, the bag and check tubes of blood.

The donated blood is positioned in coolers of ice wherein it's far stored until it is taken to the Red Cross Center.

Step Two: Processing Procedure

The check tubes are dispatched to be examined.

The Red Cross scans the blood donation into its database.

The donated blood is positioned in a centrifuge and spun to separate the transferable additives.

The Red Cross then leukocyte-reduces the crimson cells.

Platelets also are leukocyte-decreased and they're bacterially examined.

Step Three: Testing Process

There are 5 Red Cross National Testing Laboratories. The check tubes are dispatched to and then received by means of such a laboratories.

Each unit of blood undergoes a dozen exams. These tests are checking for infectious sicknesses and are supposed to establish the blood kind.

Within 24 hours, effects of the assessments are electronically sent to the producing facility.

The donor is notified if the exams return superb for infectious illnesses. The donated blood is discarded.

The checking out on this step takes place at the same time as Step two.

Step Four and Five: Storage and Distribution

Labels are placed on units of blood that undergone testing and are discovered to be safe.

Refrigerators that are kept at six levels Celsius are used for storing pink cells. Red cells are saved for forty two days simplest.

Agitators are used to shop platelets at room temperature. They are stored for not than five days.

Freezers are used to freeze and store plasma and cryo for three hundred and sixty five days.

Shipping of blood can occur at any time, seven days every week and at any hour.

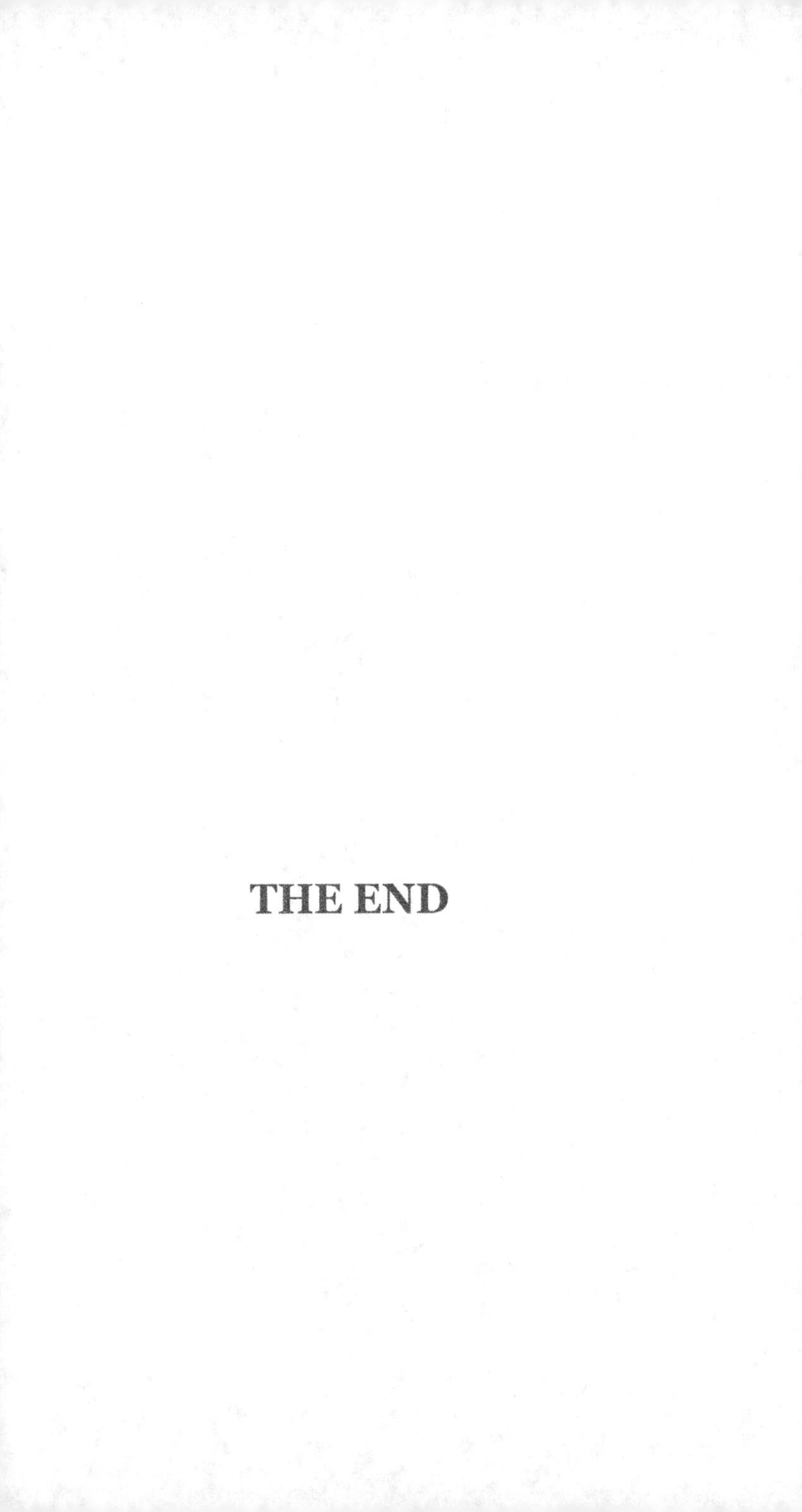

THE END